EAT RIGHT FOR YOUR HEALTHY GUM AND TEETH:

A Guide to a Healthy Smile

By

Jane Rios

Table of Content

Introduction

You are what you eat, as you've undoubtedly heard, and this is especially true when it comes to your gums and teeth.

The bacteria in your mouth that can lead to gum disease and tooth decay also enjoy starchy or sweet meals.

Your diet might make all the difference between having a healthy smile and needing frequent dental checkups. Maintaining healthy teeth over time can be challenging, even with a decent oral hygiene regimen (brushing twice a day, flossing once a day).

Healthy teeth and gums are encouraged by eating a range of

nutrient-rich foods from all the food categories. For a healthy smile and body, this means eating a balanced diet that includes fruits, vegetables, whole grains, foods high in protein, and foods high in calcium.

Chapter One:

Dietary Supplements for Strong Teeth and Gums

A healthy diet is essential to preserving the condition of your gums and teeth. A balanced diet can help ward off diseases like gum disease and cavities that can harm your teeth and gums. Eating the appropriate meals will help avoid discoloration and bad breath in addition to strengthening and protecting your teeth. Eating the correct foods and avoiding starchy, sugary, and acidic foods will help you maintain a beautiful smile and healthy teeth and gums. In this book, we'll look at how eating a healthy diet may help you maintain the health of your teeth and gums as well as how to include foods that are good in your diet.

How important is a healthy diet for gums and teeth?

Eating a balanced diet is crucial to keeping your gums and teeth healthy. Consuming the correct foods in a balanced diet will strengthen your teeth and shield your gums from diseases like gum disease and cavities. A balanced diet can supply the minerals that are necessary for strong teeth and gums, including calcium, phosphorus, and vitamin C. Eating a nutritious diet can also help you avoid tooth discoloration and maintain fresh breath.

An adequate diet for teeth and gums has numerous additional advantages. A well-balanced diet can help prevent periodontal disease by reducing gum inflammation. Tooth decay and cavities can be prevented by following a diet low in sugar and carbohydrates. Additionally, maintaining a healthy diet will strengthen your immune system generally, reducing the risk of infection in your mouth.

Can dental and oral health be enhanced by a healthy diet?

An appropriate diet can benefit dental health in several ways. Calcium, phosphorus, and vitamin C are among the vital elements that may be obtained through a balanced diet and are necessary for strong teeth and gums. Tooth decay and cavities can be prevented by following a diet low in sugar and carbohydrates. A balanced diet can also aid in reducing gum inflammation, which helps ward off periodontal disease.

An adequate diet not only supplies necessary nutrients but also helps ward off discoloration and foul breath. Eating a diet low in carbohydrates and sugary foods can help prevent tooth discoloration and lower the risk of cavities and tooth decay. Consuming a diet rich in fiber might also help lessen bad breath by naturally cleaning the teeth and gums. You are what you eat, as you've undoubtedly heard, and this is especially true when it comes to your gums and teeth.

The bacteria in your mouth that can lead to gum disease and tooth decay also enjoy starchy or sweet meals.

Your diet might make all the difference between having a healthy smile and needing frequent dental checkups. Maintaining healthy teeth over time can be challenging, even with a decent oral hygiene regimen (brushing twice a day, flossing once a day).

Healthy teeth and gums are encouraged by eating a range of nutrient-rich foods from all the food categories. For a healthy smile and body, this means eating a balanced diet that includes fruits, vegetables, whole grains, foods high in protein, and foods high in calcium.

What meals are therefore the healthiest for gums and teeth?

Fresh fruits and vegetables are some of the best foods for healthy teeth because of their high nutritional content and additional benefits for cleaning teeth. Additionally, foods high in calcium can support strong teeth and bones. Examples of these foods are low-fat or fat-free milk, yogurts, and cheese; fortified soy drinks; tofu; canned salmon; almonds; and dark green leafy vegetables. Chewing on crunchy meals stimulates saliva production, which, when combined with water, helps wash away food particles and germs that cause plaque.

Chapter Two

The Healthiest Foods for Teeth and Gum

Your food still poses a risk to your dental health, regardless of how rigorous your oral hygiene regimen is. The teeth are crucial! It makes sense that the majority of us look after them quite well. We do several things like brush, floss, scrape our tongue, and use mouthwash. Even if we may take the greatest care of our mouths, tooth decay, and gum disease remain among the most common medical conditions worldwide. Why is that? Maybe it's in the refrigerator! Unexpectedly, your diet may make the difference between having a healthy smile and needing frequent dental checkups. If you don't control what you eat, it could be difficult to maintain healthy teeth even with the best dental hygiene regimen.

Too frequently, we believe that when it comes to dental health, diet is only to blame. Ultimately, the majority of the harm done to our teeth comes from the sugars and acids found in food and beverages. But there are also a lot of food kinds that can improve your dental health and not simply cause less damage to your teeth.

The foods on this list can live up to the promises of the most expensive toothpaste and mouthwashes available, from preventing cavities and periodontal disease to even improving breath and teeth whitening. Put some teeth-friendly treats on your shopping list; the majority of them are rather tasty as well.

How certain meals maintain the health of your teeth and gums

As with any other component of your body, your teeth and gums require a healthy diet to work correctly. Let's examine which nutrients are most essential for healthy teeth and gums. Different sections of your body respond well to particular nutrients.

foods high in phosphorus and calcium

Minerals make up tooth enamel, after all. A variety of acidic meals and beverages can erode tooth enamel, thus replenishing lost minerals is necessary to strengthen your teeth again. Here, phosphorus and calcium are the key players. These are the components that makeup enamel, thus eating a diet high in them is essential to maintaining the strength and health of your teeth.

* The best sources of calcium include almonds, low-fat milk, tofu, shellfish, yogurts, and hard, aged cheese.
* The best sources of phosphorus include tofu, eggs, red meat, fish, pumpkin seeds, and Brazil nuts.

Tough, crunchy foods with lots of water

Foods that are hard, crunchy, and high in water content are beneficial to your teeth in multiple ways. First, the best natural defence against the bacteria that causes cavities is saliva, which is produced in greater quantities when you chew. Second, because of their naturally abrasive nature, these meals gently exfoliate and polish the surfaces of your teeth, eliminating food particles and plaque. This isn't an excuse to eat chips and crackers, though—it has to be raw fruits and vegetables. Top choices include carrots, apples, cucumbers, and celery.

foods high in vitamin D

Not only is vitamin D essential for good health overall, but it's also critical for dental health.* It improves calcium absorption in your body, which is the primary reason. The greatest natural sources of vitamin D are sunshine (which is the only source you can consume), salmon, egg yolks, and cod liver oil.

foods high in vitamin C

Vitamin C has great strength! It can lessen inflammation and improve blood vessels, which might keep your gums in better condition. Additionally, the synthesis of collagen—a vital protein that aids in the prevention of periodontal disease—requires vitamin C. Your gums become more sensitive and vulnerable to the bacteria that cause periodontal disease when you don't get enough vitamin C.

* The best foods include broccoli, kale, strawberries, oranges, kiwis, and bell peppers.

Antioxidant-rich foods

Antioxidants are practically celebrities when it comes to their health advantages. How do they maintain the health of your mouth? The germs that cause periodontal disease and inflammation are combated by antioxidants. They aid in preventing bacterial infection and cell damage to the gums and other tissues.

* Apples, berries, grapes, raisins, almonds, and beans are the best sources.

foods that are high in probiotics

There are a tonne of both beneficial and harmful bacteria in your body. Probiotics are among the finest, but there's already some evidence that they can support healthy gums and reduce plaque.

* The best sources include fermented foods including miso, kombucha, sauerkraut, and yogurt.

foods high in polyphenols, arginine, and anthocyanins

There are a plethora of additional factors that could improve dental health. While more research is required, some of the most promising candidates include polyphenols (which may slow the growth of bacteria leading to plaque, preventing gum disease, cavities, and bad breath), arginine (an important amino acid that may disrupt the formation of plaque and reduce chances of cavities), and anthocyanins (which may prevent the attachment of plaque on the teeth and fight oral cancer).

* The best sources of arginine are meat, soy, and nuts; * The best sources of polyphenols are tea (black and green), berries, flaxseed, cocoa, grapes, cherries, plums, and eggplant; We've already covered the reasons why diet matters for your teeth as well as some of the fundamental research underlying the relationship between oral health and nutrition. All that's left to do is provide you with a comprehensive list of some of the

healthiest meals available. So here it is!

For several reasons, cheese is considered one of the healthiest foods for teeth. It has a high calcium content and a low sugar content. It has casein, a protein that is especially helpful in strengthening dental enamel. Cheese has a lot of calcium, which is good for keeping your bones strong. Additionally, cheese has a high phosphate content, which balances the pH levels in the mouth and protects dental enamel. Cheese is also good for our teeth because it makes saliva, which helps to wash away bacteria in the mouth as we chew it.

Milk

The finest beverage for your teeth is milk, along with water. It contains a lot of calcium and other essential minerals. Additionally, milk lessens oral acid production, which aids in the prevention of tooth decay.

Water

The superhero of your teeth! Drinking water helps maintain a high salivary flow and helps wash away meal particles. Because saliva naturally fights plaque with its proteins and minerals, and because it is abundant if you drink enough water, it is your mouth's best defence against tooth decay.

Greens that are leafy (kale, broccoli, spinach)

Rich in calcium, folic acid, and other vital vitamins and minerals that are great for your teeth and gums, leafy greens are also very healthful.

Fish (wild salmon, tuna, and fatty fish)

Fish is an essential component of any diet that is tooth-friendly since it is rich in minerals and vital vitamins like vitamin D.

Meat The majority of meats have excellent dental health. They contain a wealth of the most vital nutrients that were previously stated. Particularly advantageous are red foods and even organ meats.

Green and Black Tea

Consider polyphenols! It has been demonstrated that polyphenols decrease oral bacteria and their harmful byproducts. In addition, tea usually contains a lot of fluoride, which is considered to be important for strong teeth. Drinking it sweetened won't be the best idea because even honey and sugar might spoil the festivities.

Nuts

Nuts provide numerous dental health benefits. They are brimming with vital nutrients like phosphorus and calcium. Almonds, Brazil nuts, and cashews are particularly advantageous as they aid in the fight against the microorganisms that cause dental disease.

Gum

This is an obvious choice. Chewing gum increases salivation, which removes food particles and microorganisms.

Fresh cranberries

Similar to tea, it is high in polyphenols, which prevent plaque and reduce the risk of cavities. The process of plaque development is very effectively disrupted by fresh cranberries.

Orange-coloured

Oranges are the least acidic fruit of all and offer all the health advantages associated with fruits. Most citrus fruits are highly acidic, which is bad for your teeth.

Strawberries You must adore strawberries if you desire flawless teeth! They include a wealth of antioxidants, vitamin C, and malic acid, which has the potential to naturally whiten teeth.

Yogurt

Yogurt is undoubtedly beneficial to your dental health in many ways.

Packed with probiotics and calcium, it guards against gum disease, cavities, and even foul breath.

Carrots

Carrots are delectable and a great source of many essential minerals and vitamins for your oral health, therefore they merit special attention. That Bugs Bunny has flawless teeth makes sense.

Apples

Can one apple a day prevent dental problems? Perhaps not, but it will undoubtedly be beneficial. It has many essential vitamins and nutrients.

Garlic

Garlic contains a compound called allicin, which has potent antibacterial qualities. Hence, it aids in the battle against periodontal disease in particular, and tooth decay.

Ginger

In so many ways, ginger is incredible. In terms of dental health, it may prevent the formation of bacteria and freshen your breath.

Complete grains

Eating complete grains, such as brown rice and muesli, reduces the incidence of gum disease.

Pears

Raw pears are an excellent snack at any time since, in contrast to many acidic fruits, they are adept at neutralising acids.

One of the greatest vitamin C concentrations is found in kiwis.

Onions

Onions have strong antibacterial qualities when consumed raw, notably against certain of the germs that cause gum disease and cavities.

Shiitake mushrooms

These delicious Asian treats are a plague's worst nightmare. They include lentinan, a naturally occurring sugar that prevents plaque from building up on your teeth.

Celery

Celery deserves special attention because it is very beneficial to your teeth. It is the closest thing we have to nature's floss and is, in many respects, the ideal snack for maintaining good oral health.

Soy

Soy-based diets may support the development of healthy gums.

For your teeth, Wasabi Sushi just got better! There is proof that wasabi prevents bacteria from adhering to teeth.

seeds from sesame

Rich in calcium and highly effective in removing plaque from teeth as you chew.

Sweet potatoes
Getting enough vitamin A will have a positive impact on your gums and enamel.

Raisins
This is a surprising entry because, in certain cases, raisins are even portrayed negatively regarding their impact on teeth. They do, however, contain phytochemicals like oleanolic, which have the potential to eradicate germs that cause cavities.

Antioxidants are abundant in them as well.

Never forget the fundamentals.

Eating delicious foods that you know are good for your dental health makes you feel terrific. But remember what your dentist has instructed you. It's always a good idea to clean your teeth in some way from the residual food particles, sugars, and acids, even after the healthiest entries on this list. Naturally, brushing should be your priority, but if that's not possible right now, you can at least sip some water or acquire some gum.

Chapter Three

Foods to avoid for a healthy mouth and Teeth

Since you are here, you probably know how important your oral health is for your general well-being. You are probably also aware of the value of your diet for your dental health. It seems the saying "You are what you eat" rings truer and truer and when it comes to dental health it's even more important than normal.

We've already talked at great length about what the best foods for healthy teeth and gums are in another post. Now, it's time to see what parts of your food could put your oral health in danger. Of course, most of us will never be able to eat 100% clean and remove all the "dangerous" foods and drinks from our diet, but it is important to know what to pay attention to and how to reduce the potential dangers.

We all know the name of the enemy when it comes to your teeth - plaque. We also know who plaque's bad minions are - sugar and acids. These are the main culprits as far as our mouth is concerned as they are personally responsible for enamel loss, tooth decay, and pretty much all dental problems. So, let's try to find out what types of foods and drinks are most dangerous to our mouths and hopefully, this will be a step forward for better oral health for all.

Highly Acidic Foods

When it comes to your teeth, acidic foods (foods with low Ph levels) could be extremely dangerous. Why? Whether present in foods or converted from sugars by your mouth's bacteria, acids can erode your teeth's enamel, causing cavities and tooth decay. Weakened enamel can also lead to a variety of problems ranging from sensitive issues to discoloured teeth.

Examples of highly acidic foods: are lemons, pickles, tomatoes, booze, and coffee.

Examples of low-acidic foods: are bananas, avocados, broccoli, lean meat, whole grains, eggs, cheese, nuts, and veggies.

Foods High in Sugar

We all know sugar is bad for our teeth, but it's important to know why exactly. The bad bacteria in your mouth feed on sugars to make acids and cavities are an infection caused by acids. The point here is that sugars in your mouth are often the first step in the process of cavity creation.

It's nearly impossible to eliminate all sugars from your diet, but it's important to try to minimise sugar intake (especially refined sugar) as much as possible. It's also important to not let sugar linger in your mouth for a long time. So, brushing your teeth after meals or at least drinking lots of water is important.

Examples of foods high in sugar: are sugar (duh), soft drinks, sweets, dried fruit, desserts, jams, and cereal.

Sticky/Chewy Foods

An all-star villain when it comes to your teeth and gums' health is foods that tend to stick and stay stuck to and between your teeth for a very long time. The problem is such food debris turns into a plentiful energy source for bacteria and their prolonged presence in your mouth allows bacteria to produce much more acid than usual. It's important to try to clean your teeth (flossing is best) as fast as possible and not leave sticky foods to linger in your mouth for hours.

Starchy foods and Refined Carbohydrates

Refined carbohydrates are rightly frowned upon for the many health dangers they bring. When consumed, they turn into sugars instantly in your mouth to kick-start the acid production by bad bacteria.

Many starchy foods, including white bread, potato chips, and pasta, can easily become stuck between teeth and in crevices. While you might not consider them as dangerous as sugar, it's important to note the starches begin converting to sugar almost immediately by the pre-digestive process that starts in the mouth through the enzymes in saliva.

Foods that Dry Out Your Mouth

Your best defence against oral health problems is saliva. Nature's most powerful way to take care of your teeth is to help your mouth stay healthy by washing away plaque and bringing back key minerals to your teeth. Saliva stops food from sticking to your teeth and may even help repair early signs of tooth decay, gum disease, and other oral infections. Unfortunately, when your mouth is dry, the saliva amount in your mouth gets low and it can't do its job properly.

Examples of foods and drinks that dry out your mouth excessively: are booze, some medicine, coffee, and energy drinks.

Very Hard Foods That You Chew On

Enamel is very hard. It's the hardest part of your body! However, even it can't bear you chewing often on very hard foods. It's important to remember that if something is too hard, it's not meant to be chewed.

Many people have the bad habit of chewing on ice, hard candy, and unpopped popcorn. Most of the time your teeth handle the hard job, but you can damage your enamel and there is always a danger of chipping off a piece of your teeth. So, do your teeth a favour and avoid chewing on hard objects.

Here are some dangerous Drinks and Foods for your Teeth and Gum

Soda

Nothing earns the first spot in this list as much as soda. We all know how bad soda is for pretty much all parts of our health and oral health is not an exception. A vast number of studies have shown the link between soda intake and cavities.

The danger is two-fold. First, drinks are highly acidic, and the acids found in them can harm your teeth even more than sugar by stripping minerals from your enamel. Hence, even sugar-free (diet) drinks are still pretty bad for your teeth as they contain citric and phosphoric acid. Of course, regular, sugar-containing sodas are even worse, as they have the extra danger of providing a rich sugar feast for the bad bacteria in your mouth.

Sports drinks

Even though sports drinks sound healthy, they are packed with sugar and acids and the potential for cavities and damage is very significant. A study of the erosive effect of acidic liquids on the teeth found sports drinks to be the most erosive drinks of the bunch. And that was fighting with sodas and energy drinks which are among the most acidic drinks available.

Energy drinks

The same study from above-found energy drinks to be the most acidic liquids, compared to sports drinks, sodas, and 100% juice, and the second most erosive (second to only sports drinks). So be warned that in addition to wings, energy drinks might very well give you cavities as well.

Alcohol

We know Happy Hour is the biggest reason many of us go to work on Fridays but keep in mind that all alcoholic drinks pose a serious threat to your oral health. Alcohol causes thirst and dry mouth. This reduces saliva flow which can cause major problems over time such as tooth decay and gum disease. Sipping on sugary cocktails has the added risk of bathing your teeth in sugar for a long time.

Wine

Wine gets special mention as we know it colours your teeth pretty bad and there are other dangers as well. Being an alcoholic, wine dries your mouth and can also make teeth sticky, promoting stain formation. In addition, red and white wines are very acidic which we already know is pretty bad for your teeth. Keep in mind that while red wine can damage your teeth more, white wines are more acidic, so they might be even more dangerous to your enamel.

Coffee

It's common knowledge how bad coffee stains your teeth, and coffee marks are among the worst for your teeth as they are very resistant. In addition, just like wine, coffee makes teeth sticky and also dries out your mouth. It gets even worse if you add sugar to smooth your coffee as there are few things worse for your teeth than sugar.

If that's not enough, coffee is also acidic, which we know takes down enamel. Of course, we don't expect you to stop drinking your favourite beverage, but to limit the damage please drink plenty of water afterward and try to avoid additives like sugar.

Fruit drinks

Even though not as bad as the drinks mentioned above, it's good to know most fruit juices are highly acidic and have been linked to an increased risk of cavities. Of course, 100% fruit drinks have some health benefits as well, so just be aware of their acidic nature and at least rinse your mouth with water after drinking them.

Sticky/Chewy Candy

The chances of seeing a dentist munch on toffees or other chewy candy are pretty much similar to the chances of seeing a dinosaur. The reason, of course, is doctors know how bad sticky candy is for their teeth. Their high sugar content mixed with their sticky nature makes them a nightmare for your teeth and oral bacteria's favourite snack.

Hard candy

The only thing worse than having candy trash stuck in your teeth for a long time is chipping off a piece of your tooth. If you chew hard sweets there is always a risk of damaging your enamel and in extreme cases, chipping a piece of your tooth off. So be extremely careful when chewing hard things in general.

If you don't chew hard sweets but let them melt in your mouth it might be even worse. The problem is hard candies dissolve slowly and saturate your mouth with sugar for a long time, giving bad bacteria plenty of time to make harmful acids. What's even worse, many types of hard candy are flavoured with citric acid which adds, even more, acid to your mouth.

Sour candy

Sour candy is so bad for your teeth it also gets its mention. Sour candy includes more and different kinds of acids than other varieties. What makes things worse is you can't solve the problem by brushing immediately after you eat them, because brushing too soon after consuming highly acidic foods or drinks could damage your enamel even further.

Dried fruits

Many people consider this to be a healthy snack choice and there is some value to that. However, when it comes to dental health, dried fruits mean trouble. They are filled with a big dose of natural sugars and nonsoluble cellulose fiber which makes them bad for your teeth. Your best option is to munch on fresh fruits instead.

Citrus Fruits

Yes, they are super-rich in Vitamin C and are loaded with a whole array of health benefits, but they are also loaded with acid which can eat and decay your tooth enamel. Lemon and grapefruit are the most acidic, while orange is the least acidic of the group. So if you enjoy squeezing lemons in your water and sipping on it throughout the day you might need to rethink as prolonged acid exposure is really bad for your teeth. It's better to drink or eat your lemons and then drink plenty of water to wash out the acid.

Canned fruit

Most fruits have a good amount of natural sugars in them, but canned versions are infused with lots of added sugar as well which turns them into something your teeth wished you'd avoid. Canned citrus fruit is the worst, as it mixes the very high sugar content with naturally contained acids.

Crackers

While most crackers don't contain sugars or acids and don't damage your teeth they are still pretty dangerous to your teeth. The reason is the processed carbohydrates that quickly break down into sugar! Most crackers also get gooey when you chew them, so they stick between your teeth letting bacteria grow.

Potato chips

Starchy foods get stuck between your teeth. As tasty as potato chips are, sadly, the starch in them and their mushy texture means they will stay trapped between your teeth for a long time. If possible, rinse with water and floss to remove the stuck debris.

White bread

It's refined sugars to blame again. When you chew bread the enzymes in your saliva break down the starch into sugar. Now changed into a gummy substance, the breadsticks between your teeth. To reduce the danger opt-in for whole wheat options instead.

Popcorn

We all love snacking on popcorn at the movies but beware they pose some danger to your teeth as well. First, they can get trapped between your teeth, supporting bacteria growth. Unpopped ones are nasty as they are too hard and can damage your enamel or chip off a tooth.

Peanut butter & jelly

Normally, we wouldn't dare say a bad word against most people's favourite breakfast, but the high sugar content and the stickiness of the ingredients make it a terrible choice for your teeth and a great one for the bacteria in your mouth.

Ice

It's made out of clean water, so how bad can it be? Well, it's not, unless you decide to chew it. It's a bad habit many people have, but for the sake of your teeth, please just let ice cool off your drinks and don't chew on it.

Vinegar

We use vinegar mostly in salad dressings, sauces, pickles, and some potato chips and it's important to know it can cause tooth decay. Studies have shown an increased chance of enamel erosion for people who frequently eat vinegar-containing foods. It's a crucial ingredient for a tasty salad, but you need to remember to rinse your mouth with water afterward to minimise the possible danger.

Pickles

The trouble once again is acid. Vinegar is most often the cause here. It's what gives pickles their taste and also what makes them dangerous for your teeth. We agree pickles are super tasty on your sandwich, just keep in mind they are a real teeth nightmare, and make sure to drink some water afterward to reduce the acid.

Tomatoes

Tomatoes are acidic, that's the problem your teeth have with it. Of course, if you eat them as a part of a meal, the danger is reduced. So just keep in mind that acidic foods, in general, are not very welcome by your teeth, and drink water afterward to clean your mouth.

Breath mints / Cough Drops

Fresh breath is important, but breath mints are probably not the best choice. If they stay in your mouth for a very long time, you are in effect soaking your teeth in sugar. If possible try to find sugar-free choices to minimise the danger.

They might soothe your cough, but most cough drops are filled with sugar as well. In addition, they stay in your mouth for a long time so the possibility of dental damage can be serious. Again, sugar-free solutions are better.

Tannic acid

Tannic acid can be found in drinks like red wine, coffee, and black tea. These drinks will colour your teeth and make your teeth sticky. Tannins also tend to dry out your mouth, which means your saliva levels will be dropped.

Pigmented foods

Highly coloured foods like berries, beets, and curry can easily stain your teeth. Yes, some of them are super-healthy, so please keep eating them, but you need to remember to rinse your mouth to reduce the spots.

Note: Please keep in mind that some of the foods and drinks mentioned above might have some overall health benefits as well. However, in this post, we are mostly concerned with the effect they have on your tooth health. We don't recommend eliminating all of these foods and drinks from your diet altogether. However, it's important to be aware of the possible negative effects they have on your mouth's health and know how to minimise the danger when you happen to consume them.

Chapter Four

Vitamins for strong teeth and gums

When it comes to oral health, we usually think of brushing, rinsing, and flossing as the key strategies to keep our gums and teeth healthy. However, good oral health extends well beyond this! Nutrition is critical to maintaining dental health. Teeth and bones are linked, thus all nutrients that promote bone health also promote dental health.

A vitamin and mineral-rich diet is vital for maintaining strong teeth and healthy gums. We'll look at the top ten greatest vitamins for gums and teeth and how including them in your diet can help your oral health.

Calcium

Calcium is the most abundant mineral in the body and is crucial for bone and tooth growth and maintenance. Although bones are the primary calcium storage site in the human body, teeth also require this mineral to be robust. Calcium aids in the production of dental enamel, which is required to protect your teeth from disease and erosion. Your teeth might become weak, fragile, and vulnerable to injury if you do not consume enough calcium.

Vitamin C

Vitamin C is a potent antioxidant and vitamin whose advantages extend far beyond immune health. Vitamin C can be very beneficial in maintaining healthy gums. The gums are the foundation of our teeth and must be properly nourished to be healthy. A clinical shortage of vitamin C can cause the gums to swell, become painful, and bleed easily. As a result, it's vital to take enough vitamin C in your diet to keep your gums healthy.

Vitamin D

Vitamin D is another important vitamin for tooth health. Vitamin D is a fat-soluble vitamin that aids in calcium and phosphorus absorption and metabolism. These two minerals are required by the body for the formation and maintenance of strong bones and teeth. Without enough vitamin D levels, the body cannot adequately absorb and utilise these nutrients, resulting in weakening bones and tooth decay.

Phosphorus

Phosphorus is another crucial mineral that aids in the mineralization of teeth and the creation of enamel. It works with calcium to help create and maintain strong bones and teeth. Phosphorus is the second most prevalent mineral in the body after calcium, with bones and teeth containing over 85% of the phosphorus! Phosphorus contributes to the formation of hydroxyapatite, a mineral that gives teeth their hardness and strength.

Vitamin A

Normal vitamin A levels are required to maintain healthy teeth. A lesser intake of vitamin A has been linked to poor oral epithelial growth and tooth formation. This is because vitamin A is involved in tooth growth and plays an important function in maintaining the integrity of the oral mucosa.

The vitamin K

Vitamin K is yet another fat-soluble vitamin that is vital to the health of our bones and teeth. This vitamin aids in the activation of proteins that regulate calcium levels in the body, which is necessary for strong bones and teeth. Without adequate vitamin K, our systems are unable to properly employ this mineral to maintain the health of our skeletal system.

Furthermore, persons who consume more vitamin K have higher bone density than those who do not consume enough of this mineral. This implies that getting adequate vitamin K can help prevent bone loss as we get older.

Vitamin K is essential for blood clotting in addition to its involvement in bone and tooth health.

Vitamin B

B vitamins are involved in several processes that benefit oral health, including red blood cell creation, DNA synthesis, and nerve function.

A lack of B vitamins can have a severe impact on oral health, resulting in disorders such as ulcers or mouth sores.

Potassium

There is a link between calcium and potassium consumption and oral health. This suggests that a low potassium intake is linked to tooth loss. These findings emphasise the importance of getting enough potassium in your diet.

Iron

A shortage of iron in the diet can have a severe impact on oral health, even if it does not immediately affect teeth and gums. Iron is a mineral that aids in the transfer of oxygen to the body's tissues. A deficiency of iron can cause oral symptoms such as a painful or swollen tongue and changes in tongue colour. However, it is critical to check iron levels before supplementing, as high quantities can be harmful.

Zinc

Zinc is a trace mineral that is required in enough amounts to promote healthy teeth and gums. Zinc can be found in different regions of the oral cavity, including saliva and tooth enamel hydroxyapatite. It is engaged in several processes that promote oral health, including the creation of healthy teeth and the maintenance of the oral mucosa. Because of these effects, zinc is frequently found in mouthwashes and toothpaste.

Chapter Five

Final Thought on Eating Right for Your Healthy Teeth and Gum

Foods are Meant to Make You Healthy and Happy

Other than providing you with energy, food is supposed to make you healthy and happy, so don't stress too much about what you eat as long as you follow a few basic principles that will help your teeth and gums stay healthy.

It's better to avoid substances that have an extremely negative effect on your general health (like soda), but even if you can't eat 100% clean, the following principles will help your teeth and gums stay healthier:

Your mouth needs rest, so don't munch on snacks all the time. Leave sufficient time for your mouth to heal and for saliva to naturally replenish minerals in your teeth. Keep your food intake 3-5 times a day and let your mouth rest between meals.

To lessen the danger of some of the foods and drinks on this list (and remember some of them have health benefits as well) try to consume them as part of a meal, rather than on their own.

Brushing after a meal is, of course, always a great choice. Just remember to wait 20 minutes if you've eaten highly acidic foods that have weakened your enamel.

If possible, always clean your mouth with water after a meal and drink lots of water throughout the day as well.

Use a straw when drinking highly acidic beverages to limit their contact with your teeth.

In summary, keeping optimal oral health requires a multifaceted approach that includes proper nutrition and preventative measures such as brushing, flossing, tongue scraping, and mouthwash. Vitamins and minerals play a critical role in healthy teeth and gums, making it especially important to ensure proper amounts of these nutrients through a balanced diet. Vitamin and mineral supplements can also be taken to fill any gaps in the diet or to fix any deficiencies.

Additionally, smoking cigarettes and tobacco use can have a significant negative effect on dental health, with a link between smoking and dental cavities. By incorporating healthy lifestyle choices and focusing on nutrient-dense foods, people can support optimal oral health.

Conclusion

Eating a balanced diet of the right kinds of foods can provide the important nutrients needed for healthy teeth and gums. Nutrients such as calcium, phosphorus, and vitamin C are necessary for healthy teeth and gums, and a balanced diet can provide these nutrients. Additionally, eating a healthy diet can help keep your breath fresh and avoid discoloration of the teeth. There are many other benefits to good nutrition for teeth and gums, including a well-balanced diet that can help reduce inflammation in the gums, which can help prevent periodontal disease. Eating a diet low in sugar and starches can also help reduce the chance of cavities and tooth decay. And, eating a healthy diet can help boost your general immune system, which can help protect your mouth from infection.